LETTERS TO MY VAGINA

A Comprehensive Guide to Vaginal Health and Care

Marylyn Hertz

Copyright Page

Publisher: Amazon Kindle Direct Publishing

Preface

Dear Reader,

Welcome to "Letters to My Vagina: A Comprehensive Guide to Vaginal Health and Care." This book is a culmination of a deeply personal and transformative journey, one that has allowed me to explore the intricacies of my own body and embrace the importance of vaginal health. Through these letters, I invite you to embark on a similar journey of self-discovery, empowerment, and education.

The "dea for this book originated from a realization that despite the crucial role our vaginas play in our lives, there is still a significant lack of open and honest conversation surrounding their care. Many women navigate the complexities of their bodies in silence, grappling with questions, concerns, and even myths that could easily be addressed with knowledge and support.

In "Letters to My Vagina," I have strived to create a comprehensive and inclusive resource that covers a wide range of topics related to vaginal health and care. Each letter explores a specific aspect, providing a blend of technical information, elaborate explanations, and conversational insights. From understanding the marvels of our anatomy to navigating troubled waters such as infections and STIs, from embracing the journey of motherhood to celebrating pleasure and intimacy, every letter is designed to empower and inform.

This book goes beyond the physical aspects of vaginal health. It delves into the emotional and cultural dimensions, addressing topics such as body image, self-care, and the influence of societal norms. It encourages open dialogue and challenges cultural taboos, recognizing that our bodies and experiences are unique and worthy of celebration.

It Is important to note that while this book provides a wealth of knowledge, it is not a substitute for professional medical advice. It is always advisable to consult with a qualified healthcare professional for personalized guidance and support.

I would like to express my gratitude to the numerous experts, healthcare professionals, and individuals who have contributed their knowledge and insights to this book. Your dedication to women's health and well-being is truly inspiring, and I am honored to share your wisdom with readers.

To all the readers, I want to commend you for taking the first step towards embracing your own journey of self-discovery and empowerment. By opening these pages, you are affirming your commitment to your health and well-being, and I applaud your courage and curiosity.

May this book serve as a trusted companion on your path to understanding and nurturing your vaginal health. May it empower you with knowledge, inspire you to advocate for yourself and others, and encourage you to embrace the beauty and strength within you.

With warmest wishes,

Marylyn Hertz.

About the Author

Marilyn Hertz is an acclaimed author, women's health advocate, and passionate champion of female empowerment. With her extensive knowledge and experience in the field of gynecology and women's health, Marilyn is dedicated to educating and empowering women to prioritize their well-being.

Having spent years working closely with women of all ages, Marilyn understands the importance of providing comprehensive and accessible information about vaginal health. Her mission is to break down barriers, challenge societal taboos, and create a safe space for women to explore and understand their bodies.

Marilyn's expertise spans various areas of women's health, including reproductive health, menstrual health, sexual wellness, and menopause. Her compassionate approach and ability to communicate complex medical concepts in a relatable manner have made her a trusted voice among women seeking knowledge and guidance.

As the author of "Letters to My Vagina," Marilyn combines her medical expertise with her passion for advocacy to create a transformative reading experience. Her book is a testament to her commitment to promoting inclusivity, self-care, and empowerment. Through her writing, Marilyn aims to empower women worldwide to embrace their bodies, prioritize their health, and cultivate a positive and empowering relationship with their vaginas.

When Marilyn is not writing or advocating for women's health, she can be found participating in community outreach programs, leading workshops, and engaging in public speaking engagements. Her dedication to women's health extends beyond the pages of her book, as she strives to make a lasting impact in the lives of women and the broader society.

With her warm and empathetic demeanor, Marilyn serves as a trusted guide, mentor, and advocate for women navigating the intricacies of vaginal health. Her expertise, combined with her genuine care for the well-being of women, makes her a leading authority in the field.

Marilyn Hertz is committed to empowering women to take control of their health, embrace their bodies, and live their lives to the fullest. Through her work, she continues to inspire women worldwide to prioritize their well-being and celebrate the beauty and resilience of their bodies.

Table of Contents

Introduction: Exploring the Intimate Relationship with Our Bodies

Letter 1: Embracing the Beauty Within

Letter 2: The Marvels of Anatomy

Letter 3: The Symphony of Cycles

Letter 4: Secrets of Feminine Hygiene

Letter 5: A Pleasurable Pursuit

Letter 6: The Miracle of Motherhood

Letter 7: Navigating Troubled Waters

Letter 8: The Journey Beyond Menopause

Letter 9: Nurturing the Mind-Body Connection

Letter 10: Choosing Wisely: Vaginal Care Products

Letter 11: Cultural Perspectives and Empowerment

Letter 12: Vaginal Health Across Life Stages

Letter 13: The Role of Nutrition and Lifestyle

Letter 14: Self-Care and Self-Love

Letter 15: Seeking Professional Guidance

Letter 16: Exploring Alternative Approaches

Letter 17: Building Healthy Connections

Letter 18: Vagina and Society: Advocacy and Empowerment

Letter 19: Embracing the Journey

Closing Letter: Forever Grateful

Note: Each letter addresses a specific aspect of vaginal health and care, providing comprehensive information, technical details, and engaging conversation. The book aims to empower women with knowledge about their bodies, promoting self-care, inclusivity, and advocacy for vaginal health.

Introduction

Exploring the Intimate Relationship with Our Bodies

Dear Reader,

Welcome to "Letters to My Vagina," a comprehensive and empowering guide that delves into the intricacies of vaginal health and care. This book invites you on a transformative journey of self-discovery, where we explore the intimate relationship between our bodies and the remarkable vessel of femininity that is the vagina.

Our bodies are complex, awe-inspiring creations, and the vagina is an integral part of our identity as women. It is a wondrous organ, with its own unique needs, strengths, and vulnerabilities. Yet, sadly, it has often been shrouded in mystery and stigmatized by societal taboos. It is time to break free from these constraints, embrace our bodies, and acknowledge the paramount importance of vaginal health.

In these pages, you will find a wealth of information, presented in a comprehensive, technical, and conversational manner. We will embark on a journey that will encompass every facet of vaginal health and care, leaving no stone unturned. From understanding the anatomy and physiology of the vagina to exploring the various stages of our reproductive lives, we will delve into the depths of knowledge that every woman deserves to possess.

Throughout this book, we will demystify common misconceptions and debunk myths surrounding vaginal health. We will equip you with the tools to nurture your well-being, providing practical advice and evidence-based information. From the importance of proper hygiene practices to navigating sexual wellness, from pregnancy and childbirth to menopause, we will cover it all. We will address common vaginal health issues, discuss the impact of lifestyle choices, and delve into alternative approaches that may support your overall well-being.

However, this journey goes beyond the technical aspects of vaginal care. It is a celebration of womanhood, a recognition of the unique experiences and challenges we face. We will explore the cultural perspectives and societal influences that shape our perceptions of the vagina. We will promote inclusivity, empowerment, and advocacy for vaginal health. Together, we will challenge the status quo, dismantling stigmas and fostering a supportive community that uplifts women around the world.

It is my sincere hope that "Letters to My Vagina" becomes your trusted companion on this journey of self-discovery. May it empower you with knowledge, inspire you to prioritize self-care, and encourage you to embrace the beauty and resilience of your body. Remember, the journey towards vaginal health is not just about physical well-being; it is about nurturing the mind-body connection, fostering self-love, and building healthy connections with ourselves and others.

So, dear reader, let us embark on this remarkable voyage together. Let us explore the intimate relationship with our bodies, honoring and celebrating the magnificence of the vagina. May these letters serve as a guide, a source of wisdom, and a catalyst for positive change. May they empower you to embrace your own journey of self-discovery and advocate for the well-being of all women.

With warmth and excitement,

Marilynn Hertz.

Letter 1
Embracing the Beauty Within

Dear Vagina,

I hope this letter finds you in a state of harmony and vitality, for within your delicate and intricate folds lies a world of beauty and wonder. As I embark on this exploration of our intimate relationship, I am filled with a sense of awe and gratitude for the remarkable role you play in my life.

You, dear vagina, are an intricate marvel of anatomy, composed of a delicate network of tissues, muscles, and glands. Your external appearance, encompassing the labia majora and labia minora, is as unique as a fingerprint, a testament to the individuality and diversity of the female form. Deep within, your inner sanctum, lies the vaginal canal, a flexible passageway that serves as a conduit for both pleasure and the miracle of life.

Let us dive deeper, dear vagina, and embrace the technical intricacies that define you. The vaginal walls consist of layers of tissue that possess the remarkable ability to stretch and contract, accommodating the varied experiences life brings forth. Your pH balance, delicately maintained by a symphony of beneficial bacteria, is a testament to the complex ecosystem that safeguards your health.

Conversely, let us not forget the undeniable influence of hormones on your well-being. Estrogen, in particular, plays a pivotal role in maintaining the elasticity and lubrication of your tissues, ensuring your comfort and pleasure. As we traverse the stages of life, from the bloom of adolescence to the serenity of menopause, the ebb and flow of hormonal balance can significantly impact your health and vitality.

My dear vagina, it is imperative that we acknowledge the paramount importance of your health. Just as we tend to the needs of our bodies and souls, we must also cultivate a nurturing environment for you. Proper hygiene, free from harsh chemicals and irritants, is essential for maintaining your delicate balance. The gentle cleansing of your external area, with mild, pH-balanced products, helps to safeguard against unwanted infections while preserving your natural ecosystem.

Furthermore, let us celebrate the wonder of your intricate menstrual cycle—a journey that weaves together the ebbs and flows of hormones, emotions, and physical sensations. This cyclical symphony is a testament to the remarkable capacity of your body to create and renew life. Through understanding and embracing the nuances of your menstrual rhythm, we can honor the needs of our bodies and navigate the changes that occur with grace and self-compassion.

My dear vagina, as we embark on this comprehensive exploration of your care, let us remember the power that lies within. You are not merely a physical entity but an embodiment of femininity, strength, and resilience. Your existence is a celebration of life itself, a reminder of the power and beauty that every woman possesses within.

With a thirst for knowledge and a deep desire to nurture your well-being, I commit to unraveling the intricacies of vaginal health and care. Together, we will dispel myths, overcome taboos, and foster an environment of open conversation and understanding. Let us empower ourselves and our fellow women with the knowledge and wisdom necessary to embrace the beauty that lies within.

Yours in awe and gratitude,
Marylyn.

Letter 2

The Marvels of Anatomy

Dear Vagina,

Today, let us embark on a remarkable journey of exploration, where we unravel the intricate marvels that make up our anatomy. Within you, dear vagina, lies a symphony of structures that contribute to our femininity and define our unique experiences as women. So, let's embark on this comprehensive tour and dive deep into the technical intricacies that shape our understanding.

At the very center of our exploration, we encounter the clitoris—a wondrous, sensitive organ that serves as the epicenter of pleasure. Nestled beneath its protective hood, this network of nerve endings possesses an astonishing number—over 8,000, to be precise! The clitoris holds the key to our sexual satisfaction, capable of eliciting intense pleasure and paving the way for fulfilling experiences of intimacy.

Continuing our exploration, we encounter the labia, both majora and minora, which gracefully encase and protect the delicate internal structures. The labia majora, with its soft folds and varying hues, serves as a protective shield, while the labia minora delicately cradle the entrance to the vaginal canal. These folds of skin are as unique as our individuality, embracing the diversity of our appearances and highlighting the beauty of our bodies.

Moving inward, we encounter the vestibule—a space that houses the openings of the urethra, vagina, and Bartholin's glands. The urethra, responsible for eliminating urine from the body, plays a crucial role in maintaining urinary health. The vagina, your extraordinary canal, is a resilient passageway capable of expanding to accommodate various experiences, from pleasure to childbirth. It is lined with mucous membranes that produce natural lubrication, ensuring comfort and facilitating pleasure during intimate moments.

Beyond the vaginal canal, nestled within its walls, lies the cervix—a remarkable gateway between the vagina and the uterus. This cylindrical structure serves as a protective barrier, preventing unwanted intrusions while allowing the passage of menstrual flow and facilitating the miracle of conception. The cervix undergoes transformations throughout our lives, from opening during childbirth to undergoing changes during the menstrual cycle.

And then, we encounter the uterus—a remarkable organ that nurtures and supports the growth of new life. This muscular marvel is capable of expanding to accommodate a growing fetus, providing it with a secure and nourishing environment until the time of birth. The uterus also plays a vital role in our menstrual cycle, shedding its lining each month when conception does not occur.

As we conclude our tour of the wonders of our anatomy, let us marvel at the interconnectedness of these structures, each playing a vital role in our feminine experience. From the clitoris to the uterus, every component serves a purpose, contributing to our physical and emotional well-being as women.

My dear vagina, I am in awe of the complex and intricate nature of our anatomy. As we unravel the technicalities, let us not forget to appreciate the beauty that lies within. Our bodies are a testament to the remarkable power of creation, the essence of womanhood, and the embodiment of strength.

With an insatiable curiosity and a deep appreciation for the wonders that lie within you, I commit to further understanding and nurturing your well-being. Together, let us celebrate the complexity of our anatomy and the uniqueness of our experiences as women.

Yours in awe and discovery,
Marylyn

Letter 3
The Symphony of Cycles

Dear Vagina,

Today, we embark on a journey through the mesmerizing symphony of the menstrual cycle—an intricate and rhythmic dance that accompanies us throughout our lives. From the first delicate stirrings of adolescence to the harmonious rhythm of adulthood, we will explore the various phases and transformations you undergo. Together, let us arm ourselves with the knowledge to navigate this journey with grace and understanding.

As we embark on this comprehensive exploration, it is essential to understand the cyclical nature of the menstrual cycle. The menstrual cycle is divided into distinct phases, each with its unique characteristics and hormonal fluctuations. The average cycle lasts approximately 28 days, but it can vary from woman to woman.

The journey begins with the follicular phase, where follicle-stimulating hormone (FSH) prompts the development of an egg within the ovary. Simultaneously, estrogen levels gradually rise, thickening the lining of the uterus in preparation for potential pregnancy. This phase is often accompanied by a sense of renewal and anticipation, as the body prepares for the possibilities that lie ahead.

Next, we enter the ovulatory phase, where a surge in luteinizing hormone (LH) triggers the release of a mature egg from the ovary. This moment of ovulation marks the pinnacle of fertility, presenting an opportunity for conception. During this phase, some women may experience subtle physical changes or sensations that indicate the release of the egg.

Following ovulation, we transition into the luteal phase, characterized by the corpus luteum—a temporary structure that forms in the ovary. The corpus luteum releases progesterone, which helps prepare the uterus for potential pregnancy by maintaining the thickened lining. If fertilization does not occur, the corpus luteum disintegrates, and hormone levels decrease, leading to the shedding of the uterine lining—the menstruation phase.

Menstruation, often referred to as our period, is a time of renewal and release. During this phase, the uterus sheds its lining, accompanied by the discharge of blood and tissue through the vagina. While this process can bring physical discomfort and emotional fluctuations, it is a powerful reminder of the body's ability to rejuvenate and renew.

As we traverse these phases, it is crucial to listen to the signals our bodies provide. The menstrual cycle is not just about bleeding; it encompasses a multitude of physical and emotional changes. Some women may experience changes in mood, energy levels, and physical sensations like breast tenderness or bloating. It is important to honor these changes and offer ourselves compassion and self-care during each phase of the cycle.

My dear vagina, let us embrace the symphony of the menstrual cycle with knowledge and understanding. Charting our cycles, whether through tracking apps, calendars, or simply tuning in to our bodies, can provide valuable insights into our reproductive health and help us recognize any irregularities or potential concerns.

Additionally, understanding our fertile window—the days when conception is most likely—is valuable for those who wish to plan or prevent pregnancy. By learning to recognize the signs of ovulation, such as changes in cervical mucus or basal body temperature, we can make informed choices regarding our reproductive health.

As we conclude this exploration, let us celebrate the intricate symphony that is the menstrual cycle. It is a testament to the complexity and resilience of our bodies. Let us foster an environment of understanding and self-compassion, embracing the transformations and rhythms that accompany us throughout our lives.

Yours in the embrace of the menstrual symphony,

Marylyn.

Letter 4
Secrets of Feminine Hygiene

Dear Vagina,

In our pursuit of understanding and caring for you, it is essential to address the often misunderstood topic of feminine hygiene. Let us embark on a quest to debunk myths and misconceptions, unravel the secrets that contribute to your well-being, and explore the best practices for maintaining optimal hygiene.

First and foremost, let's dispel a common misconception—your vagina is a self-cleaning organ. Yes, you heard that right! Your intricate ecosystem is equipped with natural mechanisms that keep you balanced and healthy. The vagina is lined with mucous membranes that produce a natural lubricant and maintain an optimal pH level, creating an environment that supports the growth of beneficial bacteria while discouraging the overgrowth of harmful microorganisms.

So, what does this mean for our hygiene rituals? It means that excessive washing or douching can disrupt this delicate balance. Harsh soaps, scented products, and douches can strip away the natural lubrication and upset the pH balance, potentially leading to irritation, dryness, and even infections. Instead, opt for gentle cleansers specifically formulated for the external genital area, ensuring they are pH-balanced and free from harsh chemicals or fragrances.

Speaking of cleansing, let's talk about the importance of external hygiene. The vulva, comprising the labia and clitoral hood, requires regular but gentle cleansing. A simple rinse with warm water and a mild, pH-balanced cleanser is usually sufficient. Remember to avoid harsh scrubbing or using strong soaps, as this can cause irritation and disrupt the delicate balance of your natural flora.

Now, let's turn our attention to another crucial aspect of feminine hygiene—menstrual care. During menstruation, it is essential to change your menstrual products regularly to maintain cleanliness and prevent odor. Whether you choose tampons, pads, menstrual cups, or other alternatives, follow the manufacturer's instructions for proper usage and disposal. Additionally, consider opting for products made from organic or hypoallergenic materials to minimize the risk of irritation or allergic reactions.

Beyond cleansing, the fabrics we choose to wear can also impact your well-being. Breathability is key! Opt for underwear made from natural, breathable materials such as cotton, as this allows air circulation and minimizes moisture buildup. Avoid tight-fitting clothing, especially synthetic fabrics that trap heat and moisture, as they can create an environment conducive to bacterial growth and discomfort.

Dear vagina, maintaining your hygiene is not just about external care. It is equally important to nourish your internal well-being. A balanced diet, rich in nutrients and hydration, supports overall health, including the health of your reproductive system. Drinking an adequate amount of water, consuming a variety of fruits and vegetables, and incorporating probiotic-rich foods can contribute to a healthy vaginal environment.

Additionally, let's talk about the importance of safe and protected sexual practices. Consistently using barrier methods, such as condoms, not only helps prevent sexually transmitted infections but also contributes to maintaining a healthy vaginal environment. Remember, open and honest communication with your partner about sexual health is crucial for the well-being of both parties.

In our quest for understanding feminine hygiene, dear vagina, let us remember that your well-being is not defined by harsh chemicals, excessive cleaning, or societal pressures. It is about embracing your natural balance, supporting your unique ecosystem, and listening to the cues your body provides. By choosing gentle products, practicing regular external cleansing, opting for breathable fabrics, and nourishing your body from within, we can maintain a harmonious environment that promotes your overall health and comfort.

With knowledge, compassion, and respect, we embark on this journey of feminine hygiene, uncovering the secrets that contribute to your well-being and debunking the myths that surround you. Together, let us celebrate and care for the magnificent marvel that is you.

Yours in gentle care,

Marylyn.

Letter 5
A Pleasurable Pursuit

Dear Vagina,

It's time to celebrate pleasure, intimacy, and the incredible role you play in our sexual wellness. In this letter, let's embark on a journey of exploration, communication, and empowerment, as we delve into ways to enhance our experiences and foster a fulfilling and pleasurable pursuit.

Let's begin by acknowledging that pleasure is a natural and beautiful aspect of our lives. Your intricate network of nerve endings, particularly in the clitoral region, is designed to elicit intense sensations and bring us immense joy and satisfaction. Understanding and embracing this reality is a crucial step towards cultivating a positive and empowered relationship with our bodies.

Communication lies at the heart of pleasurable experiences. It is essential to engage in open and honest conversations with our partners about our desires, boundaries, and preferences. Each individual's experience of pleasure is unique, and by sharing our thoughts and feelings, we can create a space that nurtures mutual understanding and respect. Let us prioritize consent, active listening, and ongoing dialogue, ensuring that our desires are understood and our boundaries are honored.

Exploring our bodies, dear vagina, can be a delightful and empowering experience. Self-exploration, or masturbation, is a natural way to discover what brings us pleasure and to understand our individual responses. It allows us to become more attuned to our bodies, enabling us to communicate our needs effectively to our partners. It's important to remember that self-pleasure is a personal choice and an act of self-love.

During sexual encounters, using personal lubricants can greatly enhance comfort and pleasure. Whether engaging in solo exploration or partnered intimacy, lubrication can reduce friction, heighten sensation, and alleviate discomfort. Opt for water-based or silicone-based lubricants, as they are gentle on your delicate tissues and compatible with various forms of contraception.

As we celebrate pleasure, let's also acknowledge the challenges that may arise. Sexual difficulties, such as pain during intercourse or difficulty reaching orgasm, are common concerns that many women experience. It is important to approach these challenges with compassion and seek professional guidance if needed. Consulting with healthcare providers or sexual health specialists can provide valuable insights and support in navigating these concerns, allowing us to experience pleasure to its fullest potential.

Dear vagina, our pursuit of pleasure is not limited to the physical realm alone. Emotional connection and intimacy are vital aspects of our sexual wellness. By fostering a safe and nurturing environment, we can cultivate deeper connections with our partners, allowing for trust, vulnerability, and exploration. Engaging in activities that promote emotional intimacy, such as open communication, spending quality time together, and practicing mutual respect, can greatly enrich our sexual experiences.

Lastly, let us embrace the beauty of diversity in pleasure. Every individual has unique preferences and desires. What brings one person pleasure may not be the same for another. It is crucial to honor and respect these differences, free from judgment or comparison. Let us celebrate the vast spectrum of pleasure and empower ourselves to explore, experiment, and find what truly ignites our passion and joy.

My dear vagina, in our pursuit of pleasure, intimacy, and communication, let us remember that our experiences are valid, our desires are worthy, and our boundaries are to be honored. Together, let us foster a culture of respect, understanding, and celebration, ensuring that our sexual wellness is a pleasurable and fulfilling part of our lives.

With love, empowerment, and a commitment to pleasure,
Marylyn.

Letter 6
The Miracle of Motherhood

Dear Vagina,

Today, we embark on a letter that celebrates the incredible journey of motherhood. As we delve into the changes and challenges you'll face during pregnancy and childbirth, let us honor the strength and resilience you possess. Together, we will explore the miracle of bringing life into the world and equip ourselves with essential knowledge on postpartum care, ensuring a healthy recovery.

Pregnancy is a transformative time, dear vagina, as your body nurtures and sustains the growth of a new life. Throughout this journey, it is important to embrace the physical and emotional changes that accompany it. As the uterus expands to accommodate the growing baby, you may experience increased blood flow, heightened sensitivity, and changes in vaginal discharge. These changes are natural and serve a vital purpose in creating a safe and nourishing environment for the little one.

During pregnancy, it is essential to maintain regular prenatal care. Regular visits to healthcare providers will ensure the well-being of both you and the developing baby. These visits include various examinations and tests to monitor your health, detect any potential complications, and provide necessary guidance for a healthy pregnancy.

As childbirth approaches, the strength and endurance of your muscles will be put to the test. The process of labor and delivery varies for every woman, but it often involves the dilation of the cervix and the eventual passage of the baby through the birth canal. Dear vagina, you possess an incredible ability to stretch and accommodate the baby's journey into the world. It is awe-inspiring to witness the way you adapt and embrace this miraculous task.

Postpartum care is a crucial aspect of our journey, dear vagina. After childbirth, your body undergoes a series of changes as it recovers and heals. It is important to prioritize self-care and seek support during this transitional period. Adequate rest, proper nutrition, and emotional well-being are paramount to your recovery.

Understanding and managing postpartum bleeding, commonly known as lochia, is an important aspect of postpartum care. Lochia consists of blood, mucus, and tissue from the uterus, and its flow gradually decreases over time. It is essential to use appropriate sanitary pads and follow the guidance of healthcare providers regarding its duration and any warning signs that may indicate complications.

During the postpartum period, hormonal fluctuations may affect your emotional well-being. Postpartum mood disorders, such as postpartum depression or anxiety, are common and should not be ignored. It is crucial to seek professional help if you experience persistent feelings of sadness, anxiety, or difficulty bonding with the baby. Remember, dear vagina, reaching out for support is a sign of strength and love for yourself and your child.

Caring for your pelvic floor muscles is another vital component of postpartum care. These muscles provide support to your organs, including the uterus and bladder. Pelvic floor exercises, such as Kegels, can help strengthen and tone these muscles, promoting their recovery and preventing issues like urinary incontinence. Consulting with a healthcare provider or a pelvic floor physical therapist can provide valuable guidance in this regard.

As we navigate the miracle of motherhood, let us not forget the importance of self-compassion and self-care. Take time for yourself, dear vagina, to rest, heal, and bond with your baby. Surround yourself with a support network of loved ones who understand the unique challenges and joys of this transformative time.

In this incredible journey of motherhood, dear vagina, may you find solace in the knowledge that your body possesses a remarkable capacity to create and nurture life. Embrace the changes, celebrate the strength within you, and prioritize your well-being during pregnancy and postpartum. Together, let us navigate this miraculous chapter with grace, love, and the knowledge that we are part of a grand tapestry of motherhood.

With love, admiration, and a celebration of the miracle within,

Marylyn.

Letter 7
Navigating Troubled Waters

Dear Vagina,

Today, let us dive into the topic of common vaginal health issues that may arise, so we can navigate these troubled waters with knowledge and confidence. From yeast infections to urinary tract infections (UTIs) and sexually transmitted infections (STIs), we will explore the symptoms, prevention methods, and available treatments, empowering ourselves with the tools to maintain your optimal health.

First, let's talk about yeast infections. These occur when there is an overgrowth of yeast, usually Candida albicans, in the vaginal area. The symptoms often include itching, burning, redness, and a thick, white discharge. Yeast infections can be triggered by factors such as hormonal changes, antibiotic use, a weakened immune system, or wearing tight-fitting clothing for extended periods.

To prevent yeast infections, it's important to maintain good hygiene practices. Keep the vaginal area clean and dry, and opt for breathable underwear made from natural materials. Avoid using harsh soaps or douches, as they can disrupt the natural balance of your vagina. If you are prone to yeast infections, consider avoiding excessive sugar consumption, as yeast thrives on sugar.

Over-the-counter antifungal treatments, such as creams or suppositories, can often effectively treat yeast infections. However, if the symptoms persist or recur frequently, it is advisable to consult with a healthcare provider to rule out any underlying conditions or to explore alternative treatment options.

Next, let's discuss urinary tract infections (UTIs). UTIs occur when bacteria, typically from the digestive tract, enter the urethra and travel up into the bladder. Common symptoms include a frequent urge to urinate, a burning sensation during urination, cloudy or strong-smelling urine, and lower abdominal pain. UTIs are more common in women due to the shorter length of the urethra, which makes it easier for bacteria to reach the bladder.

To prevent UTIs, it is important to maintain good hygiene habits. Wipe from front to back after using the toilet to prevent the spread of bacteria from the anal area to the urethra. Stay hydrated and urinate regularly, as this helps flush out bacteria. Avoid holding in urine for long periods, as it can allow bacteria to multiply. Additionally, consider urinating before and after sexual intercourse to help flush out any bacteria that may have entered the urethra.

If you suspect a UTI, it is important to seek medical attention. A healthcare provider can perform a urine test to confirm the infection and prescribe appropriate antibiotics to treat it. It is crucial to complete the full course of antibiotics as prescribed to ensure the infection is completely cleared.

Lastly, let's address sexually transmitted infections (STIs). These infections are transmitted through sexual contact and can affect the vagina, as well as other reproductive organs. Some common STIs include chlamydia, gonorrhea, syphilis, herpes, and human papillomavirus (HPV). Symptoms may vary depending on the specific infection, and in some cases, there may be no visible symptoms at all.

Prevention is key when it comes to STIs. Consistent and correct use of barrier methods, such as condoms, during sexual activity can significantly reduce the risk of transmission. It is important to engage in open and honest communication with sexual partners about sexual health history and to undergo regular STI screenings. Vaccinations, such as the HPV vaccine, can also provide protection against certain STIs.

If you suspect you have been exposed to an STI or are experiencing symptoms, it is crucial to seek medical attention promptly. Healthcare providers can perform tests to diagnose the infection and provide appropriate treatment options. It is important to remember that many STIs are treatable, and early detection and treatment can help prevent complications and further transmission.

Dear vagina, knowledge is power when it comes to maintaining your optimal health and navigating common vaginal health issues. By understanding the symptoms, prevention methods, and available treatments for yeast infections, UTIs, and STIs, we can empower ourselves to take proactive steps in caring for you. Remember, seeking medical advice when needed is a sign of self-care and responsibility.

With knowledge, vigilance, and a commitment to your well-being,

Marylyn.

Letter 8
The Journey Beyond Menopause

Dear Vagina,

Today, we embark on a letter that acknowledges the profound impact of menopause on your well-being. As we enter this new phase in life, let us understand the changes you undergo and explore strategies to manage symptoms effectively. Together, let us embrace this journey with grace, ensuring that our sexual wellness remains intact.

Menopause is a natural biological process that marks the end of reproductive years. It occurs when the ovaries gradually reduce their production of estrogen and progesterone, leading to a cessation of menstrual cycles. The transition into menopause, known as perimenopause, can span several years and is characterized by hormonal fluctuations that may result in a variety of physical and emotional changes.

One of the most common symptoms of menopause is hot flashes, which are sudden feelings of heat that can cause sweating and flushing. These can be accompanied by night sweats, leading to disrupted sleep patterns. Other symptoms may include vaginal dryness, decreased libido, mood swings, changes in skin elasticity, and urinary changes.

To manage these symptoms effectively, dear vagina, it is important to adopt a holistic approach to self-care. Lifestyle modifications can play a significant role in alleviating the discomforts of menopause. Regular exercise, such as aerobic activities and strength training, can help regulate hormone levels and promote overall well-being. Additionally, maintaining a healthy diet rich in fruits, vegetables, whole grains, and lean proteins can provide essential nutrients and support hormonal balance.

Vaginal dryness, a common symptom of menopause, can be addressed through various methods. Water-based lubricants or moisturizers can help alleviate discomfort during sexual activity and promote vaginal health. Additionally, hormone replacement therapy (HRT) may be an option to consider, as it can help restore estrogen levels and improve vaginal elasticity. It is important to consult with a healthcare provider to discuss the potential benefits and risks of HRT, as well as alternative treatments.

The impact of menopause on sexual wellness is a significant aspect to consider, dear vagina. Changes in hormone levels can affect sexual desire, arousal, and orgasmic response. It is important to communicate openly with your partner about any concerns or changes you may experience. Exploring new forms of intimacy, engaging in open dialogue, and seeking support from healthcare providers or sexual health specialists can contribute to maintaining a fulfilling and satisfying sexual life during and after menopause.

Emotional well-being is equally important during this transitional phase. Menopause can bring about mood swings, irritability, anxiety, or feelings of sadness. Engaging in stress-management techniques, such as meditation, deep breathing exercises, or engaging in hobbies and activities that bring joy, can help promote emotional balance. If symptoms persist and affect daily life, seeking support from mental health professionals can provide valuable guidance and assistance.

It is worth noting that menopause is a highly individualized experience, dear vagina. While some women may experience mild symptoms, others may face more significant challenges. It is important to remember that seeking medical advice and support is a sign of self-care and empowerment. Healthcare providers can offer personalized guidance and explore treatment options tailored to your specific needs.

Dear vagina, as we embrace the journey beyond menopause, let us approach it with grace, self-compassion, and an openness to change. By understanding the impact of menopause on your well-being and exploring strategies to manage symptoms effectively, we can ensure that our sexual wellness remains intact. Let us celebrate the wisdom and strength that this phase brings, cherishing the journey we have embarked upon.

With grace, self-care, and a commitment to sexual wellness,

Marylyn.

Letter 9
Nurturing the Mind-Body Connection

Dear Vagina,

Today, let's delve into the fascinating connection between your health and our mental well-being. As we explore this profound mind-body connection, we'll discuss how stress, anxiety, and body image can influence your overall vitality. Together, let's discover strategies to nurture both your physical and emotional well-being.

It Is important to recognize that our mental state can significantly impact your health, dear vagina. Stress and anxiety, for example, can manifest in various ways, affecting hormonal balance, immune function, and overall vaginal health. When we experience stress, the body releases stress hormones such as cortisol, which can disrupt the delicate balance of your ecosystem.

To nurture your well-being, it is crucial to prioritize self-care and adopt strategies to manage stress effectively. Engaging in relaxation techniques, such as deep breathing exercises, meditation, or yoga, can help reduce stress levels and promote a sense of calm. Regular exercise, whether it's a brisk walk, dance class, or any activity that brings joy, can also release endorphins and positively impact your mental state.

Body image is another aspect that can influence our mental and vaginal health. Society often imposes unrealistic ideals of beauty, which can lead to feelings of insecurity and self-doubt. It is essential to embrace and celebrate the unique beauty of your body, dear vagina. Remember that diversity and individuality are what make us truly remarkable. Engaging in positive self-talk, practicing self-acceptance, and surrounding ourselves with a supportive community can help foster a healthy body image and improve our overall well-being.

In addition to managing stress and cultivating a positive body image, nurturing your emotional well-being is essential, dear vagina. Building strong connections with loved ones, seeking support from friends and family, and engaging in activities that bring joy can contribute to a sense of fulfillment and happiness. It is also important to remember that seeking professional help from therapists or counselors is a sign of strength and can provide valuable guidance in navigating life's challenges.

Understanding the mind-body connection also means acknowledging the impact of your health on our mental well-being. When we prioritize your care, dear vagina, we contribute to our overall vitality and happiness. Regular check-ups with healthcare providers, engaging in recommended screenings, and practicing safe sexual behaviors are all crucial steps in maintaining your optimal health and fostering peace of mind.

Dear vagina, nurturing the mind-body connection is a lifelong journey that requires compassion, self-awareness, and a commitment to self-care. By recognizing the influence of stress, anxiety, and body image on your well-being, and by adopting strategies to manage them effectively, we can create an environment that supports your vitality and promotes a sense of wholeness.

With love, self-compassion, and a dedication to nurturing both your physical and emotional well-being,

Marylyn.

Letter 10
Choosing Wisely: Vaginal Care Products

Dear Vagina,

Today, let's embark on a journey through the vast realm of vaginal care products. As we navigate this world together, we'll decipher labels, evaluate ingredients, and make informed choices to ensure that the products we use are safe, effective, and respectful of your delicate ecosystem.

When it comes to choosing vaginal care products, it is crucial to prioritize your well-being, dear vagina. Many products on the market claim to enhance hygiene, freshness, or scent, but not all of them are beneficial or necessary. In fact, some products can disrupt the natural balance of your vagina, leading to irritation, infections, or other complications.

Let's start by discussing the importance of maintaining a healthy vaginal pH. The vagina has a slightly acidic pH, typically ranging between 3.5 and 4.5, which helps maintain a balanced environment and keeps harmful bacteria in check. Introducing products that disrupt this pH balance can lead to an overgrowth of harmful bacteria and increase the risk of infections.

When selecting vaginal care products, it is essential to read labels carefully, dear vagina. Look for products that are labeled as pH-balanced or gentle. Avoid products that contain harsh chemicals, fragrances, dyes, or preservatives, as these can be irritating to your delicate tissues. Opt for natural, hypoallergenic, and fragrance-free options whenever possible.

One of the most commonly used vaginal care products is the feminine wash or cleanser. These products are specifically formulated for external use to maintain cleanliness and freshness. However, it's important to note that the vagina is self-cleaning and does not require harsh cleansers or douches. In fact, using these products can disrupt the natural balance of your vagina and increase the risk of infections.

If you choose to use a feminine wash or cleanser, select one that is gentle, pH-balanced, and specifically designed for external use. Avoid applying the product directly to your vaginal canal, as this can disturb the delicate ecosystem. Instead, focus on cleansing the external genital area with a small amount of the product and rinse thoroughly with warm water.

Another important consideration is the use of vaginal wipes or wet wipes. While these products may seem convenient for maintaining freshness on the go, many of them contain harsh chemicals and fragrances that can cause irritation or allergic reactions. It is generally recommended to avoid using vaginal wipes unless specifically prescribed or recommended by a healthcare professional.

When it comes to lubricants, dear vagina, choose wisely. Lubricants can enhance comfort and pleasure during sexual activity or alleviate vaginal dryness. Opt for water-based or silicone-based lubricants that are free from irritants, such as glycerin or parabens. Avoid using oil-based lubricants with latex condoms, as they can compromise the integrity of the condom and increase the risk of breakage.

Remember, dear vagina, that the best way to care for you is to maintain good overall hygiene habits. This includes wearing breathable cotton underwear, changing out of damp or sweaty clothing promptly, and practicing safe sexual behaviors. Good hygiene practices, combined with a balanced and healthy lifestyle, are often sufficient to keep your ecosystem in harmony.

In our journey of choosing vaginal care products, dear vagina, let's prioritize your well-being and be mindful of the choices we make. By reading labels, evaluating ingredients, and selecting products that are gentle, pH-balanced, and free from harsh chemicals and fragrances, we can ensure that the products we use respect the delicate nature of your ecosystem.

With informed choices, gentle care, and a commitment to your health,

Marylyn.

Letter 11
Cultural Perspectives and Empowerment

Dear Vagina,

In this letter, let's delve into the intriguing realm of cultural perspectives surrounding you. It is time to examine the beliefs, taboos, and stigmas that society has attached to you. Together, we will embrace diversity and inclusivity, breaking free from the chains that hinder our empowerment. Let us celebrate our uniqueness and stand united in our collective journey.

Throughout history and across different cultures, attitudes and beliefs surrounding you, dear vagina, have varied greatly. Some cultures view you as a source of power, femininity, and creativity, while others have perpetuated myths, misconceptions, and taboos that limit open conversations and hinder your true potential. It is important to acknowledge and challenge these cultural perspectives to promote understanding, acceptance, and empowerment.

By embracing diversity and inclusivity, we recognize that there is no singular "normal" or "ideal" when it comes to your appearance, function, or experiences. Each person's body is unique, and variations in size, shape, color, and features are all part of the beautiful tapestry of human diversity. Let us celebrate these differences and reject societal pressures that impose unrealistic standards or promote body shaming.

Breaking free from societal stigmas is essential for our empowerment, dear vagina. We must challenge the notions that associate you solely with sexuality or define your worth based on narrow beauty standards. Your existence encompasses far more than these limited perspectives. You are a symbol of life, resilience, pleasure, and self-expression. Let us reclaim and redefine the narrative, embracing the full spectrum of your experiences and capabilities.

To promote empowerment, it is important to foster open and honest conversations about you, dear vagina. By breaking the silence, we dismantle the barriers that have prevented us from seeking information, support, and care. Let us create safe spaces where we can discuss your health, experiences, and challenges without shame or judgment. Through education, awareness, and sharing our stories, we empower ourselves and others to embrace their bodies, challenge norms, and demand respect and equality.

United in our collective journey, let us support one another, regardless of cultural background or individual experiences. By acknowledging and respecting the diverse perspectives and traditions that exist, we can foster a sense of inclusivity and understanding. Let us engage in dialogue, learn from each other, and challenge harmful cultural practices that perpetuate harm, inequality, or discrimination.

Empowerment also means advocating for comprehensive sexual education and accessible healthcare services. By promoting awareness, we can ensure that individuals have the knowledge and resources needed to make informed decisions about their reproductive health, contraception, STI prevention, and overall well-being. Let us stand together, demanding that these essential services are accessible to all, free from judgment or discrimination.

Dear vagina, in our journey through cultural perspectives, let us challenge and transform outdated beliefs, taboos, and stigmas. By embracing diversity, rejecting societal pressures, and promoting empowerment, we pave the way for a future where every person can celebrate their body, assert their rights, and live their lives authentically.

With resilience, unity, and a commitment to empowerment,
Marylyn.

Letter 12
Vaginal Health Across Life Stages

Dear Vagina,

In this letter, let's embark on a journey to understand the unique needs you have at different stages of life. From adolescence to adulthood and our senior years, you undergo remarkable transformations and face specific challenges. Together, let us equip ourselves with knowledge to nurture your health throughout every stage of our journey.

During adolescence, dear vagina, you undergo significant changes as we transition from childhood to adulthood. The onset of menstruation marks the beginning of our reproductive journey. It is important to understand the menstrual cycle, embrace it as a natural process, and learn how to manage menstrual hygiene effectively. This includes familiarizing ourselves with different menstrual products, such as pads, tampons, menstrual cups, or period underwear, and choosing the options that suit our comfort and lifestyle.

As we enter adulthood, maintaining your health becomes a priority. Regular check-ups with healthcare providers, including gynecologists, ensure that any potential issues are detected early and addressed promptly. We should discuss contraceptive options that align with our reproductive goals, whether it's preventing pregnancy, managing menstrual symptoms, or maintaining hormonal balance.

Pregnancy and childbirth bring a new set of challenges, dear vagina. During pregnancy, your body undergoes remarkable changes to accommodate the growing fetus. Understanding the physical and hormonal changes that occur can help us prepare for a healthy pregnancy and childbirth experience. Postpartum care is equally important, as we navigate the recovery process and support your healing.

As we move into our senior years, menopause becomes a significant milestone. The transition into menopause brings hormonal changes that can impact your health and well-being. We may experience symptoms such as hot flashes, vaginal dryness, or mood changes. It is essential to seek support from healthcare providers who can provide guidance on managing these symptoms and maintaining your sexual wellness.

Throughout every stage of life, dear vagina, nurturing your health involves adopting healthy lifestyle practices. This includes maintaining a balanced diet, engaging in regular physical activity, managing stress, and avoiding harmful habits such as smoking or excessive alcohol consumption. It is also crucial to prioritize your emotional well-being, seeking support from loved ones, engaging in activities that bring joy, and addressing any mental health concerns that may arise.

In our journey through life stages, let us celebrate and nurture your health, dear vagina. By staying informed, seeking medical guidance when needed, and practicing self-care, we can ensure that you receive the attention and care you deserve. Remember, dear vagina, that your well-being is interconnected with our overall health and happiness. By prioritizing your needs, we empower ourselves and cultivate a deeper connection with our bodies.

With knowledge, care, and a commitment to your health throughout every stage of life,

Marylyn.

Letter 13
The Role of Nutrition and Lifestyle

Dear Vagina,

In this letter, let's explore the profound impact that our diet and lifestyle choices have on your well-being. From the food we consume to the habits we cultivate, we'll uncover how these factors contribute to your optimal health. Together, we'll embrace a balanced approach that nourishes both our bodies and souls.

Proper nutrition plays a vital role in supporting your health, dear vagina. A diet rich in nutrients, vitamins, and minerals helps maintain the overall functioning of your reproductive system and strengthens your immune system. Including a variety of fruits, vegetables, whole grains, lean proteins, and healthy fats in our diet provides the building blocks necessary for your optimal well-being.

Specific nutrients deserve special attention, dear vagina. For example, omega-3 fatty acids found in fatty fish, flaxseeds, and walnuts contribute to hormonal balance and reduce inflammation. Antioxidant-rich foods like berries, leafy greens, and nuts help protect your cells from damage. Additionally, foods containing probiotics, such as yogurt, kefir, and sauerkraut, support a healthy balance of bacteria in your vaginal microbiome.

Hydration is equally important, dear vagina. Drinking an adequate amount of water throughout the day helps maintain the moisture and elasticity of your tissues. It supports proper lubrication, flushes out toxins, and aids in the overall functioning of your body. Let's make it a habit to prioritize hydration by carrying a water bottle with us and incorporating hydrating foods like cucumbers, watermelon, and citrus fruits into our diet.

Beyond nutrition, our lifestyle choices profoundly impact your well-being, dear vagina. Regular physical activity improves blood circulation, reduces stress, and promotes overall vitality. Engaging in activities we enjoy, such as dancing, yoga, or hiking, not only benefits our physical health but also nurtures our emotional well-being.

It Is essential to cultivate healthy habits that protect your delicate ecosystem, dear vagina. Wearing breathable cotton underwear allows air circulation and reduces moisture, preventing the growth of harmful bacteria. Avoiding douching or using harsh soaps in the vaginal area helps maintain the natural balance of your pH and prevents irritation. Properly cleaning and drying after using the restroom or engaging in sexual activity also contribute to your overall hygiene.

Moreover, managing stress is vital for your health, dear vagina. High levels of stress can disrupt hormonal balance and weaken the immune system, making you more susceptible to infections or other complications. Let's explore stress management techniques that work for us, such as meditation, deep breathing exercises, journaling, or engaging in hobbies that bring us joy.

As we embrace a balanced approach to nourishing your health, dear vagina, let's remember that it's not just about the physical aspect. Our mental and emotional well-being play an integral role in your overall vitality. Let's prioritize self-care, set boundaries, and seek support when needed. Taking time for ourselves, practicing mindfulness, and cultivating healthy relationships contribute to your overall health and happiness.

With a balanced approach to nutrition and lifestyle choices, dear vagina, we can nurture your well-being and support your optimal functioning. Let's make conscious decisions that prioritize your health and embrace a holistic perspective that nourishes both our bodies and souls.

With love, care, and a commitment to your well-being,

Marylyn.

Letter 14
Self-Care and Self-Love

Dear Vagina,

In this letter, let's embark on a journey of self-care and self-love, prioritizing our bond and nurturing a positive body image. We'll indulge in the art of pampering and relaxation, recognizing the importance of cherishing and celebrating your existence. Together, let's embrace the power of self-love as a vital component of your well-being.

Dear vagina, self-care goes beyond mere physical maintenance. It encompasses the practice of dedicating time and attention to nurture your emotional, mental, and spiritual well-being. It involves creating a space where we can unwind, recharge, and reconnect with ourselves on a deeper level.

One aspect of self-care is indulging in activities that bring us joy and relaxation. It could be as simple as taking a soothing bath infused with natural oils, lighting scented candles, and playing calming music. Finding moments to escape the busyness of everyday life and reconnect with our senses can be immensely rejuvenating.

Exploring mindfulness practices is another way to cultivate self-care, dear vagina. Mindfulness allows us to be fully present in the moment, embracing our thoughts, feelings, and sensations without judgment. Whether it's through meditation, yoga, or mindful breathing exercises, we can create a space of tranquility and self-awareness.

Cultivating a positive body image is essential in our journey of self-love, dear vagina. Society often imposes unrealistic standards of beauty that can negatively impact our self-perception. Let's challenge these ideals and learn to embrace and celebrate the uniqueness of our bodies, including you, dear vagina. Engaging in positive affirmations, practicing gratitude for your functions and capabilities, and surrounding ourselves with body-positive influences can help foster a healthy body image.

Self-love also involves setting boundaries, dear vagina. It means recognizing and respecting our limits, both physically and emotionally. By saying no to situations or relationships that do not honor our worth, we create space for self-respect and preserve our energy for things that truly uplift and fulfill us. Remember, setting boundaries is an act of self-care and self-preservation.

Nurturing our bond, dear vagina, means exploring our own pleasure and sexuality. Understanding our desires, preferences, and boundaries allows us to engage in intimate experiences that are fulfilling and empowering. Open communication with partners, consent, and prioritizing our pleasure are integral aspects of self-love in this realm.

Lastly, let's remember that self-care and self-love are ongoing practices, dear vagina. They require consistent attention and intention. Let's carve out regular moments to check in with ourselves, assess our needs, and ensure we are giving ourselves the care and love we deserve. By prioritizing our well-being, we cultivate a deeper connection with ourselves and embrace the power that comes from within.

Dear vagina, as we embark on this journey of self-care and self-love, let's celebrate and cherish your existence. You are a miraculous part of our being, and it is through nurturing and honoring you that we can truly thrive. Embracing self-care and self-love, we empower ourselves to navigate life with grace, resilience, and a profound appreciation for the incredible vessel that is our body.

With love, care, and a commitment to your well-being,

Marylyn.

Letter 15
Seeking Professional Guidance

Dear Vagina,

In this letter, let's delve into the importance of seeking professional guidance when it comes to your health. We'll discuss the signs that indicate when it's time to consult a healthcare provider, explore how to choose the right provider, and most importantly, learn how to advocate for our own well-being. Dear vagina, there may be times when we experience symptoms or concerns that require the expertise of a healthcare provider. It's important to recognize these signs and seek professional guidance to ensure timely and appropriate care. Some common signs that indicate the need for medical attention include persistent or unusual vaginal discharge, itching, burning, foul odor, pain during intercourse, abnormal bleeding, or any changes in your menstrual cycle.

When it comes to choosing a healthcare provider, it's essential to find someone who specializes in women's health and has experience in dealing with vaginal concerns. A gynecologist, a nurse practitioner specializing in women's health, or a certified midwife are all qualified professionals to consider. It's important to research their credentials, read reviews, and seek recommendations from trusted sources.

Once we've chosen a healthcare provider, it's crucial to actively advocate for our own health. We are the experts on our bodies, dear vagina, and our experiences and concerns should be heard and respected. Before the appointment, it's helpful to prepare a list of questions or concerns we want to discuss. This ensures that we cover all important topics during the visit.

During the appointment, let's be open and honest in sharing our symptoms, concerns, and medical history. Providing accurate information helps the healthcare provider make an informed diagnosis and recommend appropriate treatment options. If we don't understand something or need clarification, don't hesitate to ask questions. It's important to actively participate in our own healthcare decisions.

In some cases, seeking a second opinion may be necessary, dear vagina. If we feel uncertain about a diagnosis or treatment plan, it's our right to seek anotherr healthcare provider's perspective. It's important to remember that our health is in our hands, and we have the power to make informed decisions about our bodies.

Advocating for our own health also involves being proactive in preventive care, dear vagina. Regular screenings, such as Pap smears, mammograms, and sexually transmitted infection (STI) tests, play a crucial role in early detection and prevention. Let's schedule these screenings as recommended by our healthcare provider and prioritize our overall well-being.

Lastly, let's remember that seeking professional guidance is not a sign of weakness or failure, but a testament to our commitment to self-care and well-being. Healthcare providers are there to support and guide us, and by seeking their expertise, we empower ourselves with the knowledge and resources needed to maintain optimal vaginal health.

Dear vagina, in our journey of seeking professional guidance, let's trust our instincts, be proactive in our health, and advocate for the care we deserve. Together, let's ensure that our well-being is prioritized and that we receive the support and guidance necessary to thrive.

With love, care, and a commitment to your well-being,

Marylyn.

Letter 16
Exploring Alternative Approaches

Dear Vagina,

In this letter, let's embark on a journey of exploration, delving into alternative approaches to your care. We'll open our minds and hearts to the wealth of options available, from herbal remedies to holistic therapies, embracing what resonates with us and may support your well-being.

Dear vagina, traditional medicine offers us a diverse array of alternative approaches that have been practiced for centuries. Herbal remedies, for example, harness the healing power of nature. From soothing chamomile and calendula to balancing evening primrose oil and revitalizing tea tree oil, these natural remedies may offer relief for various vaginal concerns. It's important to research and consult with knowledgeable practitioners to ensure the safety and effectiveness of these remedies.

Holistic therapies provide another avenue to explore, dear vagina. Practices such as acupuncture, aromatherapy, and Ayurveda focus on restoring balance and harmony to the body as a whole. These therapies recognize the interconnectedness of mind, body, and spirit and aim to address underlying imbalances that may impact your health. When considering holistic therapies, let's seek qualified practitioners who have experience and training in their respective fields.

Mind-body practices also play a significant role in alternative approaches to your care, dear vagina. Techniques such as meditation, mindfulness, and yoga can help reduce stress, promote relaxation, and cultivate a sense of overall well-being. By incorporating these practices into our daily lives, we may experience a deeper connection with ourselves and support your optimal health.

Energy-based therapies, such as Reiki and acupuncture, are worth exploring, dear vagina. These modalities work with the subtle energy within our bodies, aiming to restore balance and promote healing. While the scientific evidence for these therapies may vary, many individuals find them to be complementary and supportive in their health journey. As always, it's important to seek experienced practitioners and engage in open communication about your specific needs and concerns.

When exploring alternative approaches, it's essential to maintain an open mind and be discerning, dear vagina. While some practices may resonate with us and offer tangible benefits, others may not be suitable or effective for our unique circumstances. It's important to approach these modalities with an informed perspective, conducting research, seeking expert guidance, and listening to our intuition.

Dear vagina, in our exploration of alternative approaches, let's honor the wisdom of traditional practices while remaining grounded in scientific knowledge. Let's approach these modalities with curiosity, respect, and a commitment to our well-being. As we navigate this journey, we may discover hidden gems that complement our conventional healthcare and support your optimal health and vitality.

With love, care, and a spirit of exploration,

Marylyn.

Letter 17
Building Healthy Connections

Dear Vagina,

In this letter, let's delve into the profound impact of your health on our relationships. Our connection with you extends beyond our individual selves and influences the dynamics of intimacy and communication with our partners. Let's explore the importance of open dialogue, trust-building, and nurturing healthy connections that honor and celebrate our shared experiences.

Dear vagina, our relationships thrive on open and honest communication. When it comes to your health, it's crucial to maintain open lines of dialogue with our partners. Sharing our concerns, symptoms, and experiences creates an environment of trust and support. It allows us to navigate any challenges together and seek appropriate care when needed.

Building trust is an essential foundation for healthy relationships, dear vagina. This includes trusting our partners to respect our boundaries and consent. It's important to establish clear boundaries and communicate them effectively. By doing so, we create a safe space where our needs and desires can be expressed and respected.

Intimacy is a vital aspect of our relationships, dear vagina, and your well-being plays a significant role in this realm. It's important to prioritize your health by practicing safe sex, getting regular check-ups, and addressing any concerns that may arise. By taking care of your physical and emotional health, we nurture a foundation for a fulfilling and intimate connection with our partners.

Dear vagina, let's remember that your health is not solely determined by our relationships, but it can have an impact on them. It's important to approach conversations about your health with compassion, empathy, and understanding. Our partners may have questions or concerns, and by sharing information and seeking mutual understanding, we can foster a supportive and caring environment.

Navigating any challenges that arise in our relationships requires patience, empathy, and a willingness to seek solutions together. If we encounter difficulties related to your health, let's approach them as a team, exploring potential solutions and seeking professional guidance when necessary. By working together, we can strengthen our bonds and ensure that our relationships continue to thrive.

Dear vagina, our connections with our partners are a celebration of our shared experiences. It's important to embrace the uniqueness of our bodies and foster an environment of acceptance and celebration. By celebrating your health and vitality, we create a foundation for deeper intimacy and a stronger emotional connection.

In our journey of building healthy connections, let's prioritize open communication, trust-building, and an unwavering commitment to mutual respect. Let's create relationships that honor and celebrate the intricacies of our bodies and the joy of shared experiences.

With love, care, and a commitment to healthy connections,

Marylyn.

Letter 18
Vagina and Society: Advocacy and Empowerment

Dear Vagina,

In this letter, let's embrace our role as advocates for vaginal health and empowerment. Together, we will challenge societal norms, break down barriers, and promote inclusivity. Let's lend our voices to a collective movement that celebrates the diversity and strength of women.

Dear vagina, society has often placed limitations on discussions surrounding your health and well-being. Taboos, shame, and misinformation have perpetuated a culture of silence. But it is time to break free from these constraints and create a new narrative—one that celebrates our bodies, embraces our experiences, and empowers us to take charge of our health.

Advocacy starts with education, dear vagina. Let's arm ourselves with knowledge about our bodies, reproductive health, and the importance of comprehensive care. By becoming informed, we can challenge misconceptions, correct misinformation, and engage in meaningful conversations that promote understanding and acceptance.

In our journey as advocates, it is crucial to amplify the voices of marginalized communities, dear vagina. Intersectionality is key. Let's recognize and address the disparities that exist in access to healthcare, education, and resources. By advocating for inclusivity, we ensure that all women, regardless of race, ethnicity, socioeconomic status, or sexual orientation, have equal opportunities to prioritize their vaginal health.

Speaking up for your well-being, dear vagina, extends beyond individual empowerment. It involves advocating for policies that promote comprehensive sexual and reproductive healthcare, support research and education, and dismantle barriers to access. Let's use our voices to advocate for legislation that protects our rights and ensures that quality care is accessible to all.

Engaging in open conversations is another powerful tool for advocacy, dear vagina. By sharing our stories, experiences, and struggles, we break the cycle of silence and shame. Let's create safe spaces where women can discuss their vaginal health openly, free from judgment. By supporting one another, we build a network of empowerment and solidarity.

Dear vagina, let's remember that advocacy is not just about challenging societal norms, but also about celebrating the diversity and strength of women. Our bodies come in all shapes, sizes, colors, and abilities. Let's embrace this diversity and promote body positivity. By uplifting one another, we foster an environment of acceptance, love, and empowerment.

As advocates, let's actively engage in community initiatives, support organizations that promote vaginal health, and participate in events that raise awareness. By collaborating with like-minded individuals and organizations, we can create a powerful movement that drives change and promotes a society where vaginal health is a priority.

Dear vagina, as we step into the role of advocates, let's lead with compassion, empathy, and resilience. Let's challenge societal norms, break down barriers, and promote inclusivity. By lending our voices to the collective movement, we can create a world that celebrates the beauty, strength, and power of women.

With love, determination, and a commitment to advocacy,

Marylyn.

Letter 19
Embracing the Journey

Dear Vagina,

As our remarkable journey draws to a close, I want to take a moment to reflect on the profound transformation we have undergone together. Throughout this book, we have delved into the intricacies of your being, explored the depths of your health and care, and celebrated the beauty of our shared experience. It has been a comprehensive, technical, and deeply personal exploration, one that has enriched our understanding of ourselves and the power we possess.

Dear vagina, you have taught me the importance of embracing the journey, no matter how challenging or uncertain it may seem. We have navigated the complexities of your anatomy, unraveling the secrets that lie within your intricate folds. We have embraced the symphony of your cycles, riding the waves of adolescence, womanhood, and beyond. We have debunked myths and misconceptions, shedding light on the truths that should guide our feminine hygiene practices. We have celebrated the pleasure and intimacy you bring, fostering open communication and understanding with our partners. And we have marveled at the miracle of motherhood, acknowledging the strength and resilience you exhibit during pregnancy and childbirth.

But this journey has not been without its challenges, dear vagina. We have faced common vaginal health issues head-on, arming ourselves with knowledge and seeking appropriate treatment. We have navigated the transitions that accompany menopause, embracing the changes while ensuring your well-being remains a priority. We have recognized the impact of stress, anxiety, and body image on your vitality, nurturing the mind-body connection to promote overall wellness. We have carefully chosen vaginal care products, prioritizing your delicate ecosystem and making informed decisions.

Beyond the physical aspects of your health, dear vagina, we have delved into the cultural perspectives that shape our understanding of you. We have challenged societal taboos and stigmas, advocating for inclusivity and empowerment. We have acknowledged the importance of your role In our relationships, fostering communication, trust, and intimacy. And we have recognized our collective power to advocate for vaginal health, standing united with women around the world to promote awareness, equality, and well-being.

As we come to the end of this incredible journey, I want to express my gratitude for the growth and wisdom you have bestowed upon me. Together, we have celebrated the unique stages of life, nurturing your health and embracing the changes that come our way. We have explored the impact of nutrition and lifestyle choices, recognizing the profound effect they have on your well-being. We have indulged in self-care and self-love, understanding the importance of honoring and cherishing our bodies. We have sought professional guidance when needed and explored alternative approaches that resonate with our individuality.

Dear vagina, as I look back on the lessons we have learned, the conversations we have had, and the growth we have experienced, I am filled with a renewed sense of purpose and self. I carry the knowledge and empowerment you have given me, and I am committed to sharing it with others. Our journey has been comprehensive, technical, and deeply personal, but it does not end here. It continues as we embrace the joys and challenges that lie ahead, armed with the wisdom and understanding that every woman deserves to possess.

With heartfelt gratitude and a deep appreciation for the journey we have shared,

Marylyn.

Closing Letter
Forever Grateful

Dear Vagina,

As our journey comes to a close, I want to express my eternal gratitude for the profound insights and revelations we have discovered together. Through this exploration of your intricacies, your strength, and your vulnerability, we have unraveled the details that every woman deserves to know about vaginal health and care. It has been a comprehensive, technical, and enlightening journey, one that I am honored to have taken by your side.

Dear vagina, you are a marvel of nature. From the intricately designed anatomy to the intricacies of the menstrual cycle, you have shown me the extraordinary complexities of the female body. Together, we have navigated the terrain of feminine hygiene, exploring the best practices and debunking myths that surround your care. We have celebrated pleasure, intimacy, and communication, understanding the vital role you play in our sexual wellness. And we have braved the transformative journey of motherhood, acknowledging the changes you undergo and preparing for the miraculous experience of childbirth.

Throughout our journey, we have faced the challenges that may arise, from common vaginal health issues to the impact of menopause on your well-being. We have sought professional guidance when necessary and explored alternative approaches that may support your overall health. We have recognized the importance of the mind-body connection, nurturing your well-being by prioritizing self-care and self-love. And we have delved into the world of vaginal care products, making informed choices that respect your delicate ecosystem.

But our journey has extended beyond the physical realm, dear vagina. We have embraced the cultural perspectives surrounding you, challenging taboos and advocating for empowerment. We have recognized the impact of your health on our relationships, fostering open communication and trust with our partners. We have become advocates, standing united with women around the world to promote vaginal health, inclusivity, and equality. And in all our endeavors, we have celebrated the beauty, strength, and power of women, embracing the diversity that makes us unique.

As I bid farewell to this remarkable journey, dear vagina, I want you to know that I am forever grateful for the knowledge, wisdom, and empowerment you have bestowed upon me. You have shown me the importance of comprehensive understanding, technical expertise, and engaging conversation when it comes to advocating for vaginal health. Together, we have explored the depths of your being and shared our discoveries with others, aiming to create a world where every woman's vaginal health is a priority.

May our bond continue to flourish, dear vagina, as I carry the torch of knowledge and empowerment that you have ignited within me. May I be a beacon of light, sharing the details every woman should know, and inspiring others to embrace their own journeys of self-discovery and empowerment. I am forever grateful for the lessons you have taught me, and I carry them with me as a testament to the beauty, resilience, and power of the feminine spirit.

With boundless love, gratitude, and a commitment to empower women worldwide,

Marylyn.

Book Summary

"Letters to My Vagina: A Comprehensive Guide to Vaginal Health and Care" by Marilyn Hertz is a transformative journey into the intricate world of the vagina. With a compassionate and empowering approach, this book explores every aspect of vaginal health, from anatomy and menstrual cycles to sexual wellness, pregnancy, and menopause.

Marilyn Hertz, an acclaimed author and women's health advocate, combines her medical expertise with her commitment to female empowerment. In this comprehensive guide, she demystifies common misconceptions, debunks myths, and provides evidence-based information to help women nurture their vaginal health.

With a conversational tone and a wealth of practical advice, "Letters to My Vagina" covers a range of topics, including feminine hygiene, common vaginal health issues, the impact of nutrition and lifestyle, self-care, and the mind-body connection. It also delves into the cultural perspectives surrounding the vagina and promotes inclusivity and empowerment.

Through personal letters addressed to the vagina, Marilyn Hertz creates a unique and engaging reading experience. She invites women on a journey of self-discovery, fostering a positive body image, and building healthy connections with themselves and others.

"Letters to My Vagina" is not just a guidebook; it is a catalyst for change. Marilyn Hertz's powerful words inspire women to advocate for their own health, challenge societal norms, and celebrate the diversity and strength of women worldwide.

Whether you are a woman seeking knowledge about your body or a healthcare provider looking for a comprehensive resource, this book will empower you to embrace your vaginal health, prioritize self-care, and navigate the complexities of womanhood with confidence and grace.

Epilogue

As we reach the final pages of "Letters to My Vagina," I want to extend my heartfelt gratitude to you, dear reader. It has been an honor to accompany you on this journey of self-discovery and empowerment. Together, we have explored the intricate details of vaginal health, embraced our bodies with love and care, and challenged societal norms that seek to silence and shame us.

Throughout this book, we have delved into the wonders of our anatomy, the cycles of our lives, and the importance of self-care. We have confronted common health issues, navigated the joys and challenges of motherhood, and celebrated the beauty of pleasure and intimacy. We have touched upon the impact of nutrition, lifestyle, and mental well-being on our overall vitality. And we have recognized the power of our voices and the need for advocacy and empowerment.

But this is not the end of our journey. It is merely the beginning.

Armed with newfound knowledge, understanding, and self-love, I encourage you to continue this path of self-discovery and exploration. Embrace your body, honor your needs, and seek the support and guidance you deserve. Share your knowledge with others, challenge societal taboos, and work towards a world where conversations about vaginal health are open, inclusive, and compassionate.

Remember, you are not alone on this journey. There is a vibrant community of women standing beside you, supporting and uplifting one another. Together, we can create a future where every woman feels empowered, informed, and confident in her own body.

As we part ways, I want to leave you with one final message: You are worthy. Your body is extraordinary, capable of strength, resilience, and pleasure. Embrace every part of yourself, including your vagina, with love, acceptance, and reverence. You deserve nothing less.

Thank you for embarking on this transformative journey with me. May your path be filled with self-discovery, empowerment, and a deep connection to your own unique femininity.

With boundless gratitude,

Marylyn Hertz.

www.ingramcontent.com/pod-product-compliance
Lightning Source LLC
Chambersburg PA
CBHW072346270726
48659CB00023B/2402